Getting a Good Night's Sleep

Sam Wesley

Sleep disorders are common in modern life and in no small measure have been caused by the things we do to ourselves. We eat too much, causing overweight, we take too many medicines, we work too hard, we party too long. The net result is that we don't get enough sleep.

Finally, we expect too much, of ourselves and of others. This contributes to our stress and our sense of failure, and exacerbates our sleeping problems.

The personal, social and economic costs are enormous, but usually the cause is not appropriately identified. Dealing with these problems is easy, providing a correct assessment has been made. This book should be a starting point in self-awareness and management.

Introduction

I am increasingly aware that the majority of my patients complain of some trouble sleeping – be it poor sleep, unrefreshing or broken sleep, or daytime tiredness.

The problem is apparent in a wide range of individuals, from those suffering pain or stress to those experiencing acute psychiatric disturbance. It seems to me that these people have little hope of getting well if their most basic needs are not being met. How can anyone meet the challenges of life if they are not sleeping well and are constantly tired?

This book seeks to share some of the findings and insights I have gained over the years from scientific literature, books and colleagues - but most importantly from my patients. It is dedicated to everyone who wants to get a good night's sleep, not just now and then but as a matter of course.

Sleep well.

Why Sleep?

We sleep for one-third of our lives and yet amazingly little is known about why we sleep. Since the time of the Ancient Greeks, philosophers and scientists have tried to unlock the mysteries of sleep but no one has been able to explain it satisfactorily.

There are many theories, but that is all they are. Aristotle proposed that after food was ingested it evaporated into gases that caused sleep. Anthropologists claim that sleep was organized around the day-time availability of hunted food, or for self-preservation by avoiding being hunted.

Sigmund Freud theorized that sleep is a way of returning to the womb, fulfilling the need for warmth and comfort. Other theories suggest that sleep is vital for acquiring memories and learning skills, for developing neural pathways in the brain and maintaining the immune system.

These theories may explain the functions and benefits of sleep, but we still don't know why we need to be unconscious for these functions and benefits to occur: as we all know, a rest just doesn't cut the ice.

How much sleep do we need?

The answer to this question depends mainly on our age, although it can vary considerably between people of the same age. Margaret Thatcher has claimed she was a four hours a night sleeper and Thomas Edison is reported to have said that his three-hour sleeps were merely a bad habit. These people are, however, exceptional: most adults find they require at least eight hours of uninterrupted sleep to avoid fatigue, irritability and a drop in performance.

Babies sleep about 17 hours a day, but by the time the baby is a year old this comes down to 14 hours. By the age of five most children sleep for 12 hours. Most elderly people sleep less, and find their sleep may be broken, particularly if the nap during the day.

In elderly people 'deep sleep' is reduced by 60 per cent and the number of arousals in the night doubles. People over 70 spend more time in bed but less time asleep.'

The quality of sleep

During deep sleep, growth hormone, which plays a vital role in the repair and maintenance of bodily tissues and the immune system, is released. If we don't get enough quality sleep we may be prone to colds and viruses. Quality of sleep can be impaired by drugs, alcohol, nicotine, caffeine, extremes of temperature, noise, stress, pain and snoring.

How many people have sleep problems?

According to British and American sleep researchers, insomnia affects between 15 and 30 per cent of the population. This means it must rank close to the top of the list of common health complaints.

Sleep loss

Like food and water, sleep is vital for our good health. Sleep loss can be cumulative and result in increasing sleep debt. Estimates suggest that in the US most people sleep one to one and a half hours less than they need. During a regular five-day working week this can accumulate to a seven-and-a-half-hour sleep debt.

If you are sleep-deprived your behavior will be similar to that of an intoxicated person. Symptoms of sleep loss include:

• Slowed reaction time.

• Impaired decision-making and faulty judgment.

- Reduced ability to concentrate.
- Difficulty with hand-eye co-ordination.
- Susceptibility to minor illness.
- Low motivation.
- Less attention to detail.
- Increased sensitivity to pain.
- Increased irritability and lower stress tolerance.

Most sleep problems are the result of an overactive mind, tension, stress, body-clock difficulties and bad sleep habits. Sleepy people are everywhere - driving cars, looking after children, operating machinery. Some problems are short-lived, but many people become chronically sleep-deprived and can become a hazard to themselves and the community.

Lack of sleep is not a trivial problem. Sleep-deprived individuals have told me the real consequences of being tired. I have two children whom I love dearly. They demand my full attention and I do find that when I am tired I shout at them. They haven't done anything wrong - they're just being kids. I wish I didn't lose my temper with them. I hate myself for that. I feel as if
I am setting a bad example when I shout. I can't help it - everything gets on top of me. When I sleep well I am so much more in control and I am sure I am a better mother.
Josie, 37

My husband and I have demanding jobs as well as a family. We are often tired. If I don't sleep properly I get very scratchy and so does he. Our sex life has been going down the tubes. We are too tired to be bothered. I hope we can get our marriage back on an even keel.

Anna, 43

If I am honest I had been partying hard - lots of late nights. I think I am an eight or nine hours a night sleeper usually but I had only been sleeping for five or six hours per night for most of the week. By the time Saturday came I was tired. I was driving to the shops at about three in the afternoon when I fell asleep at the wheel of my car, drove off the road and was stopped by a lamp post. I have since discovered that people have a body-clock dip in the middle of the afternoon so I suppose my accident was the result of driving when my body was at its lowest ebb as well as sleep loss.

Drew, 24

I am a nurse and my work is very demanding. I often work long hours and I am a shift worker. Sometimes I don't know how to keep going. I thought that even if I was tired I could still cope - that was until I gave someone the wrong medication. It could have been disastrous. I gave myself a scare.

Julie, 28

I haven't slept well for months - I have had a stressful period in my life. Not sleeping has made me tired and I have become run down. I caught the flu weeks ago but just when I am getting over it I seem to get knocked back again: I just can't shake it off. If only I could sleep better my health would improve and I would feel on top of things to sort out some stressful situations. Mark, 55

Sometimes sleep loss is just inconvenient, but bigger problems can arise. We may become irritable, which in turn destroys relationships; and it can be a health and safety hazard, ranging from small incidents to, sadly, loss of life itself.

Key points

• We all vary in the amount of sleep we need. Most adults require about eight hours.

• Up to 30 per cent of the population has a sleep problem.

• Lack of sleep causes deterioration in all human activities and can be dangerous.

• The quality of sleep we get is as important as the quantity of sleep.

What Happens When We Sleep

A patient recently explained to me that at bedtime he felt sleepy and relaxed but could not find the 'sleep switch'. It was an interesting analogy, but in fact sleep does not work like a lamp: it is not either 'on' or 'off'. Sleep has two quite distinct elements, non rapid eye movement and rapid eye movement sleep.

Non rapid eye movement sleep

During non rapid eye movement (NREM) sleep, your physical and mental activities slow down. NREM sleep is divided into four stages. When you go to sleep, you start with stage one, when you are easily roused and you can hear what is going on around you, and progress through stages two and three to the deep sleep of stage four.

Most deep sleep occurs within the first four hours.

Stage 1: Eyes roll slowly from side to side, although not as rapidly as in REM sleep.

Stage 2: All bodily functions decrease; breathing and pulse slow down and blood pressure drops.

Stage 3: Brain waves become larger and slower.

Stage 4: Body temperature drops.

Young children have considerably more deep sleep than adults. It is almost impossible to wake some children when they are in the night's first stage of deep sleep. In adolescence deep sleep decreases by about 40 per cent, and by the time we are 60 deep sleep is probably no longer present .

Rapid eye movement sleep

Rapid eye movement (REM) sleep is when you do most of your dreaming. It occurs at the end of each sleep cycle (see Figure 1). The majority of REM occurs during the first four hours of sleep.

REM is in fact a very busy time. Those of you who have watched a cat or dog sleep will attest that it isn't just their eyes that move rapidly - the whole body can twitch. In REM sleep the brain is extremely active and you dream. During dreaming the brain 'disconnects' the major muscles so that we don't act out our dreams

(which is lucky for some of us!).

During REM sleep:

• eyes move rapidly about 80 per cent of the time;
• breathing, pulse and blood pressure become irregular;
• muscles twitch, especially toes and fingers;
• erections may occur;

• brain waves are irregular and resemble those of a person who is awake.

An interesting theory about dreaming is that the dreamer is scanning the environment for threatening signs. If everything is safe, sleep continues and external noises are incorporated into dreams; if the environment is not safe the sleeper wakes.

REM sleep and dreaming enhance our ability to cope with emotional problems, so it's easy to see why it's important not to miss out on this type of sleep.

If you are sleep-deprived you may experience the 'REM rebound', in which a mass of REM is condensed early on in the sleep. This has its down side: too much REM in one go can be tiring.

The sleep cycle

A normal sleep pattern starts with NREM stage one sleep followed by stages two, three and four, and then REM sleep. The process of going through these stages is known as a sleep cycle. There are usually four or five sleep cycles during the night, each lasting about one and a half hours (see Figure 1).

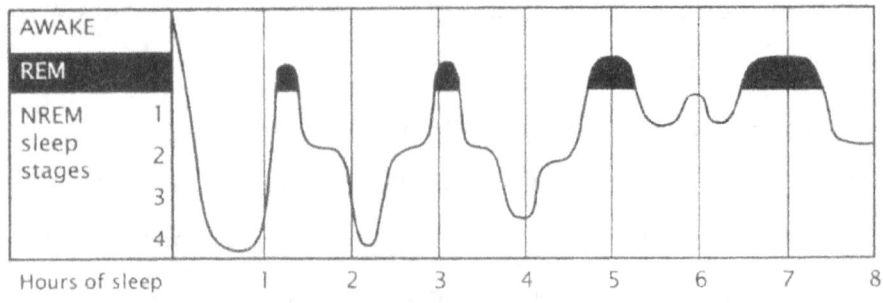

Figure 1: Sleep cycles

The body clock

All living creatures have a natural biological rhythm, or body clock, in which physiological changes occur in yearly, monthly or daily cycles. The daily rhythms of sleeping, waking and eating are the ones we are most aware of. All daily rhythms are known as the circadian rhythms (from the Latin circa, about, and dies, day).

The body clock is not related to biorhythms, which are thought to be cycles of creative, intellectual and physical activity. Although the biorhythm theory is highly plausible, it is not embraced by the scientific community.

The body clock regulates the timing of bodily functions: it tells us when to sleep, eat, rest and be active. You might think that it would take 24 hours for the body clock to go through its cycle, but in reality for most of us the clock runs slow, at about 25 hours.

If we were left to freewheel - to sleep, eat and be active when we felt like it without the cues of daylight and darkness, clocks and regular daily activity - we would go to bed an hour later each night and get up an hour later the following day.

In order to keep us in sync with the earth's 24-hour clock we depend on external cues known as zeitgebers to keep us on track, the dominant one being light and dark. Thomas Edison (the same man who could get by on three hours' sleep a night!) rendered this zeitgeber less effective when he invented the electric light bulb.

Most of us now maintain the 24-hour rhythm society demands by disciplining ourselves to go to bed at about the same time each night and getting up at about the same time each morning.

Key points

• Sleep is an active process.

• Sleep is divided into REM (rapid eye movement) and NREM (non rapid eye movement). NREM is further divided into four stages.

• REM is important for our mental health and NREM for our physical health.

• The body's internal clock runs on a daily or circadian rhythm which co-ordinates our bodily functions to meet the demands of everyday life. It tells us when to sleep, eat, be active and when to rest.

Sleeping Disorders

If you have trouble sleeping you may wonder if you have a serious sleeping disorder, and you will certainly want to know how to relieve the problem. You probably want to know what types of treatments are available: should you see a counselor, a homoeopath, a doctor, an acupuncturist, a hypnotist? Should you stop drinking coffee? Should you try relaxation techniques? Would ear plugs help?

But first things must come first, and the most important thing to do is to get an accurate assessment of the sleeping problem. This chapter will provide you with a summary of the sleeping disorders people most commonly seek help for, to help you work out what type of sleeping problem you have and what course of action you can take.

If you are in any doubt, speak to your doctor.

Insomnia

By far the most common sleeping difficulty is insomnia, literally meaning 'without sleep'. If you suffer from insomnia you may feel you hardly sleep at all - although sleep researchers have found that the majority of insomniacs lose less sleep than they think they do.

Worrying about lack of sleep and inaccurately assessing how much we sleep is quite common. I worked with one young man who told me that he never slept - he said he would just lie awake at night, tossing and turning. He had tried everything to help him sleep, but nothing worked. Eventually he underwent an assessment at a sleep laboratory, which showed that he actually slept about five hours each night. He was a lot happier when he discovered this, stopped obsessing about his sleep and, not surprisingly, once he stopped worrying he started sleeping more.

Insomnia is associated with a variety of physical and psychological causes, including disruption of the sleep-wake cycle because of shiftwork or travel across time zones, stress, depression, pain and consumption of alcohol and caffeine.

The three main types of insomnia

• Initial insomnia - difficulty getting to sleep at bedtime. This might be because you are nervous and worried, or have an excessively busy mind.

• Interrupted insomnia - waking up during the night. This often happens when there is a medical problem involving pain or respiratory difficulty. Alternatively, it may be that you have inadvertently taught yourself to wake during the night.

• Early morning awakening - waking up too early. Most often this is the result of a shifted body clock (circadian rhythm), but it can also be a warning sign for depression.

SLEEPING DISORDERS do so. The body can only last without breathing for a few minutes before damage may occur to the brain and vital organs of the body.

When the sleeper breath-holds, the body's defense mechanisms are alerted by the drop in oxygen levels in the blood and stimulate the brain to wake the sleeper.

In severe cases this can occur everyone to two minutes. The sleeper will usually be unaware of the awakenings themselves but the symptoms can be marked:

• day-time sleepiness;
• morning headaches;
• memory lapses;
• breathlessness;
• remarkably quick sleep onset (similar to narcolepsy);
• heartburn;
• waking unrefreshed;
• drop in libido.

Management

• First manage any medical disorders with the help of a medical professional.
• Use the strategies for sleep outlined in Chapter 4.
• Address the underlying psychological and stress issues.

Sleep apnoea

People with this condition hold their breath during sleep. Literally translated, apnoea means 'without breathing'. There has been a growing awareness over recent years of the health and safety hazards of sleep apnoea, the most serious of which is the increased risk of dying during the night. If you have sleep apnoea, you should be aware that taking sleeping pills is potentially dangerous.

I asked a respiratory physician why he was interested in sleeping disorders, and he told me that when he was a junior doctor one of his patients had died in her sleep simply because she stopped breathing.

He vowed to make sleep a safer place, and today he runs a sleep laboratory where he assesses and treats people who suffer from sleep apnoea. Many of his patients come to the clinic at the request of a concerned partner - the patient's main complaint is bruised ribs from their bedfellow digging them in the ribs and shouting, 'Don't forget to breathe!'

Typically, the spouse of the person with sleeping apnoea notices that their partner snores loudly and seems to stop breathing for anything up to a minute. Breathing has stopped because the throat is blocked - the sleeper makes increasing efforts to breathe but cannot do so. The body can only last without breathing for a few minutes before damage may occur to the brain and vital organs of the body.

When the sleeper breath-holds, the body's defense mechanisms are alerted by the drop in oxygen levels in the blood and stimulate the brain to wake the sleeper.

In severe cases this can occur everyone to two minutes. The sleeper will usually be unaware of the awakenings themselves but the symptoms can be marked:

• day-time sleepiness;
• morning headaches;
• memory lapses;
• breathlessness;

• remarkably quick sleep onset (similar to narcolepsy);

• heartburn;

• waking unrefreshed;

• drop in libido.

On their own these symptoms may not appear too serious, but if you suffer from sleep apnoea you are more likely to have a motor vehicle accident as a result of falling asleep at the wheel. Those most at risk are men, especially as they grow older and when they have been drinking, if they are overweight and have 'thick necks'. The first line of treatment for sleep apnoea is likely to be weight loss and reduction of alcohol consumption. However, women, young people and thin people can also suffer from sleep apnoea.

Management

If you have mild symptoms you can help yourself by:

• losing weight;

• reducing your alcohol intake;

• reducing sinus problems using asthma and allergy medication;

• stopping or reducing the use of sleeping pills;

• using a mouth splint designed to hold your jaw in place and maintain an open airway;

• improving lung function by stopping smoking and by controlling respiratory disorders.

Moderate to severe symptoms may require:

• Continuous Positive Airway Pressure (CPAP), a mechanical device consisting of a face mask with a generator that consistently pumps air into your mouth and nose to prevent collapse of your upper airways muscles;
• surgery to maintain an unobstructed airway, for example, enlarging your throat or clearing your nasal passages.

Abnormal body movements in sleep

Many of us jerk our limbs as we fall asleep. These movements may increase when we are under stress, but they do not require treatment.

Some types of body movements can disturb sleep (of either the person who is twitching or their bed partner), and therefore need attention.

Periodic leg movement syndrome (PLMS)

The toes and sometimes the whole leg twitch and jerk throughout the night. The constant movement can disrupt your sleep patterns and so cause day-time sleepiness. Some doctors think that PLMS is caused by kidney failure or vitamin deficiency, but often the cause is not identified.

Restless leg syndrome (RLS)

If you have RLS (sometimes known as 'nervous legs') you feel irritation in your legs while you are awake, making it hard to relax enough to fall asleep. The feeling may be of crawling skin or of pins and needles under the skin. The cause is not certain, although some doctors believe it is due to poor circulation - and it seems to get worse with age.

Management

• Moving relieves the discomfort of RLS. Some people find stretches or leg exercises help.
• Exercise during the day to help relax the muscles at night.
• Clonazepam, a prescription tranquillizer, can be useful.

Teeth grinding

Night-time teeth grinding, or bruxism, is usually picked up by dentists who notice their patients' teeth are blunt. Dentists have found evidence of teeth grinding in up to 20 per cent of the population. It seems to run in families and is made worse if you overdo the alcohol or have too much stress in your life. The main concerns about bruxism are day-time tiredness, headaches caused by jaw tension, and excessive wear and tear on the teeth.

Management

• A dentist may give you a mouth guard to protect your teeth.

• Address underlying anxiety by relaxation training, counseling or psychotherapy.

Bad dreams

Sometimes referred to as abnormal sleep behaviors, there are two types of bad dream.

Night terrors

Most parents have been woken by a child shrieking in the middle of the night, sitting up as if shocked by some dreadful vision.

Fortunately the terror is rarely remembered in the morning. Most children grow out of night terrors and generally no treatment is required.

Occasionally night terrors continue into adulthood. People have been known to get up and leave the house while asleep, so the most important part of management is keeping the person safe. One thing worth noting is that night-time screamers frighten parents and spouses much more than they do themselves. It is rarely the screamer who complains! Night terrors are not a sign that there is anything seriously wrong.

Nightmares

We all have nightmares from time to time but some of us have recurrent nightmares or themes that can be upsetting. A nightmare is really an anxiety dream. If you are troubled by nightmares you may find you have other difficulties, such as headaches, migraines and stomach problems. Closer investigation may reveal you have had an emotional upset, with feelings of hurt and anger. The only effective management is to address the underlying issues, perhaps with the help of a counselor.

Body clock shifts

Phase shifts

I have seen several people who can't get to sleep until the early hours of the morning. In the morning they are understandably tired, so they sleep in until late. Given the opportunity, they would go to bed later each night and get up later each morning. Teenagers and students who do not have set bedtimes and getting up times are especially prone to shifts in their body clock.

In itself this sleep disorder, called a circadian shift, is not a problem except that it puts you out of sync with most of society. It is probably more of a problem to parents than teenagers!

Management

• Go to bed at a regular time.

• Get up at a set time every morning regardless of how tired you are.

• When possible go out in the sun during the day to help set your body clock to day-time alertness and night-time tiredness.

• Do not have day-time sleeps.

• Use very bright light (see page 26) to artificially adjust your body clock.

Jetlag

Jetlag is the disruption to sleep and the feeling of fatigue you have when you fly across time zones. It is caused by confusion of your body clock. The situation is made worse by the less than comfortable flying environment: dehydration, stale air, cramped conditions and lack of exercise make it difficult to sleep on the plane, not to mention overeating, increased coffee and alcohol intake, and nicotine withdrawal if you are a smoker on a non-smoking flight.

Symptoms of jetlag include:

• tiredness during the day;

• disorientation/confusion;

- lack of energy;
- broken sleep after arrival;
- loss of appetite;
- frequent night-time urination;
- decreased concentration.

It takes one day for every time zone crossed to fully recover from jeglag, so if, for instance, you travel from England to New Zealand it takes 12 days to fully adjust to the new time zone. To maximize adjustment you need to minimize the effects of flying and help your body clock adjust to the new time zone.

Management

- During the flight drink plenty of water to keep hydrated, walk up and down the aisle to ease muscle tension and minimize swelling of the feet, and be moderate with food, alcohol and coffee.

- On long-haul flights take a sleeping pill to minimize sleep debt. I am not usually in favour of them, but the benefits of using prescription sleeping pills on long flights outweigh the dangers. A sleeping pill on the first night in your destination will help you to initiate a new sleep-wake cycle. Sleeping pills often cause drowsiness the next day, so they should not be used if alertness is required soon after arrival.

• Homoeopathic supplements are designed to alleviate anxiety, muscle soreness, stress, insomnia and dehydration. They work only on the side-effects of flying - they do not claim to shift the body clock.

• One proven way to shift the body clock is the use of bright light.

Ensure that you receive as much bright sunlight as possible in your new time zone. If you are a regular traveller you could investigate bright light therapy.

• As soon as you arrive, "live in accordance with the new time zone: eat breakfast at the new breakfast time, lunch at the new lunchtime, go to bed at the new bedtime, and so on.

• If you feel sleepy during the day (which is likely to occur at bedtime in your home country), do your best to stay awake. Instead go for a swim or take a walk (see the nine switches of alertness.

• If your trip is brief it may be easier to keep your body clock scheduled to 'home time'. It can, however, be disconcerting to your hosts if you decide to eat your evening meal at 1 a.m. and go to bed at 6 a.m.!

Shift work

If you have a job that requires you to work during the night and sleep during the day, the constant body clock shifts may wreak havoc with your sleep patterns. The problems associated with shift work can be serious, and are fully covered in Chapter 10.

Narcolepsy

People who have this condition suddenly and for no reason fall sound asleep. It can happen during a conversation, at work, driving a car. It can happen several times a day, lasting for anything from a few minutes to over an hour. It can be embarrassing if it happens to you at a dinner party, costly in a business meeting, and fatal while driving.

Other symptoms include sudden muscle weakness causing you to collapse (cataplexy). These attacks are often triggered by stress or laughter. Some patients experience sleep paralysis, which means that on falling asleep or waking they feel literally paralyzed. Some people with narcolepsy describe a strange phenomenon in which they dream while awake, causing confusion between dreams and reality.

Usually there is a family history of narcolepsy. Males are affected slightly more often than females. The age of onset varies from childhood to middle age but most typically the first narcolepsy experience happens during the late teens or early twenties.

Some symptoms are similar to those of sleep apnoea (see page 9).

It is important you get a correct diagnosis because, although there is no known cure for narcolepsy, apnoea can be treated very effectively. If you have narcolepsy you need to think in terms of managing symptoms in order to live as full and active a life as possible.

Management

• Educate your family and your employer about symptoms and management.

• Adapt your work and social life to avoid activities where falling asleep might put you or others at risk.

• Minimize sleep debt by making sure you get the right amount of uninterrupted sleep every night.

• Take strategic 'power naps'.

• Avoid occupations that interfere with your body clock, for example, jobs that require shift work or international travel.

• Exercise.

• Reduce your alcohol intake, or cut it out altogether.

• Talk to your doctor about taking a prescription stimulant to minimize day-time sleepiness.

• Join a support group.

Key points

• There are a variety of causes of poor sleep: medical, psychological and emotional.

• Insomnia is the most common sleeping disorder and there are different types of insomnia.

• Your management plan will depend on the correct assessment of the cause of your sleep problem.

• Medical conditions need to be treated as a priority.

Sleep Retraining

Most of us have a sleepless night from time to time but some people find it hard to return to good sleeping habits. Many of those who sleep badly have actually 'taught' themselves to do so. This may sound unlikely - who would want to lose sleep? - but it is usually inadvertent. The good news is that you can just as easily turn the situation to your advantage, and teach yourself to sleep well.

The strategies in this chapter work well with the majority of people I have treated and, best of all, using them will mean a good night's sleep without resorting to drugs and other sleeping aids.

Changing the messages

The way we behave is for the most part a direct response to what's going on around us. We respond to stimuli - many of them objects which have become associated in our minds with thoughts, feelings and behavior. For example, when you hold a pen you know how to write with it; when you pick up the telephone you listen and speak.

You do not have to think about what to do with these objects, because they prompt certain behavior from you. This is because you have been speaking into telephones and using pens for years, so what they do and how you use them is programmed into your subconscious.

This is a useful skill because with it you save time and energy. Anyone who has recently learned to drive a car will know how difficult and tiring it is when you have to concentrate on every action: changing gear, looking in the mirror and using the clutch. It is all so much easier for an experienced driver, who automatically knows how to drive a car because it is programmed into the subconscious.

The theory that how we behave can be affected by the objects around is known as Stimulus Control Theory, and it is a useful one for people with sleep problems. Changing the message we receive from an object is called stimulus control therapy. Consider the messages you receive from your bed and your bedroom. If every time you think of your bedroom you think about sleep, comfort, happiness and relaxation, you are probably a good sleeper. If you associate your bedroom with thinking, planning, worrying, studying or just lying awake, the chances are you have sleep problems. If the messages you receive from your bed are about not sleeping it will be necessary to teach yourself new messages. Purists would go so far as to say that in order to sleep well we should use the bedroom only for sleep and sex (although that doesn't mean that you can't have sex in other places!).

Getting the wrong message from an object is surprisingly common. Gavin was studying for his university exams. He found that often when he sat at his desk to study he would fall asleep. As soon as he woke up he would say to himself, 'I must be tired, I'd better go to bed.' Once he got into bed, though, he would perk up again and decide to go back to studying. For Gavin the message from bed was 'Study!' The message from his desk had become 'Sleep!' Life had become confusing, but Gavin was able to retrain himself to associate his desk and bed with study and sleep respectively.

For some the bedroom is associated with distress and the message is one of trauma. Betty had been abused by her husband, and the emotional and physical pain she had endured in the bedroom was so great that bad memories flooded her when she even thought about her bedroom. She went to counseling and decided to go and stay at her sister's house, where she felt secure, until she felt ready to face the past. Peter's path turned out to be much easier. He enjoyed his work as an accountant, was happily married, loved life and had minimal stress, but still when he went to bed he would toss and turn and stay awake. He had learned to associate his bed with being awake. He learned to break this association by getting up and doing something.

He had tried this technique before, but had fallen in to the trap of doing something he enjoyed or doing some work. This acted as a reward for being awake: he had started to teach himself that not sleeping at night could be pleasant or useful.

The key for Peter was to get up and do something boring and not useful. (The up times should be about 20 minutes long. If when you return to bed you are still awake after 20 minutes, repeat the procedure.)

When Marjorie went to bed she enjoyed listening to phone-in shows on the radio. When she wanted to go to sleep she turned the radio off. If she couldn't get to sleep she would turn the radio back on. She was inadvertently associating her bed with stimulating discussion and was rewarding herself for staying awake. Once she employed the 'sleep and sex only' rule she was sleeping normally within three weeks. She still enjoys radio phone-ins, but makes sure she listens to them in a different room.

Jan and Steve have two children and work long hours. Often the only time they could talk was in bed at night. The bedroom became the place where they planned their week, talked about money matters, their children, holidays - in fact anything important was discussed at bedtime. These conversations made their minds active and not surprisingly they both started to find it difficult to go to sleep.

They recognized the problem themselves and had considerable success with the following plan.

• They go for a walk once a week to spend time together and discuss matters that affect them at home.

• They set aside time to address money issues and pay the bills.

• They make the bedroom a sanctuary, a place for sleep and sex only.

Staying out of bed

Many insomniacs go to bed early. Their theory is this: it is going to take hours to get to sleep so they need to go to bed early to make time for the long hours of wakefulness. It may seem perfectly logical, but they will probably end up sleeping less. Sleep restriction therapy involves spending less time in bed. You start off spending the amount of time in bed that you know you can sleep. For example, if you typically spend 8 hours in bed but only sleep for 4 hours, you would start off by spending only 4 hours in bed. The time in bed gradually increases until you get adequate sleep.

Jane found that by going to bed later, she felt more ready for sleep and managed to sleep soon after going to bed. She devised the following plan with considerable success.

• She went to bed later at night - and got up earlier in the morning (at first she planned to be in bed for five hours).

• She delayed her getting-up time by another half hour every three days.

• When she was getting up in the morning at the time she wanted to (7.30 a.m.) she started adjusting her bedtime until she built up her time in bed to between eight and nine hours.

It wasn't plain sailing, but at the end of a month she was sleeping normally - a huge achievement for someone who had slept badly for years. She put her success down to sticking to a system, and using relaxation techniques (see pages 22-25). She realized she was sleeping badly because she expected to sleep badly: she was making

a self-fulfilling prophecy. Restriction therapy helped her to sleep when she was in bed - and success brought with it a new belief, that sleep was possible. Sleep became easier and easier once she believed in her ability to sleep. She still had the odd sleepless night, but she coped by reminding herself that it is normal to have the occasional bad night.

Sleep affirmations

Some of us can only sleep in perfect conditions - in other words there has to be complete silence. If you are one of these people, the chances are you were the first born in a family, with parents so worried about waking you when you were a baby that they made sure noise was kept to an absolute minimum. Unfortunately in doing this they taught you that perfect sleep can be achieved only in perfect conditions. Parents with more than one child soon learn to change this philosophy, and subsequent children are taught to sleep with any amount of noise going on around them. If you need perfect sleeping conditions (which of course are rarely obtained) you can teach yourself to sleep through noise using an affirmation, which you silently repeat to yourself before you go to sleep.

I will sleep deeply and easily throughout the night.

This affirmation worked very well for Rosie, a 50-year-old woman with three grown-up children. She described herself as a light sleeper: the slightest noise would wake her up. She lived in a busy suburban area where nocturnal noises were constant, and to make matters worse her husband was a snorer. Using the above affirmation she taught herself to wake up only if she needed to. She even learned to sleep through her husband's snoring.

Fran, an elderly woman who was kept awake by her husband's snoring, needed a different sort of affirmation. The problem was that not only did he snore but he had sleep apnoea, which meant that he held his breath as well. When her husband was breath holding
Fran would lie awake, worrying about whether he would start breathing again.

It was important to send Fran's husband to a sleep clinic to treat his sleep apnoea, and to reaffirm to Fran that she would wake up if her husband had a serious breathing problem. Her affirmation was:

I will sleep easily throughout the night and will only wake up for health or safety reasons.

The ability to tune in only to specified noises when sleeping is extremely useful. Among my patients are people who have taught themselves to be quite specific about what they hear, including a mother who listens to hear her baby breathing, a yachtsman who listens to hear the sound of the anchor dragging, and a motorcyclist who listens for the sound of footsteps near his precious Harley
Davidson. These people only hear what they need to hear and tune everything else out.

Changing the way we talk

High achievers and perfectionists, people who drive themselves hard, who feel they have to get things done and do them well, are high on the list of people likely to develop insomnia. If you fit into this category it may help to change the words you use and the way you talk.

Perfectionists often use the phrases 'must', 'should have' and 'got to', words they first heard from parents and schoolteachers. As adults they may not have teachers and parents telling them what to do, but many talk to themselves using the same language. The result is they feel pressure, stress, and physical and mental tension; and if they rebel, they usually feel guilty afterwards. Ultimately there is a drop in performance - leading to more feelings of failure and yet more pressure. It is hardly surprising that so many high achievers don't sleep well, with all this on their minds.

By changing the way we talk to ourselves, we can change the way we see the world and what we think of as the world's expectations of us. If we can see that we do have choices we can start to feel more in control. The Greek philosopher Epictetus put it perfectly when he said, 'Man is not disturbed by events but the view he takes of them.'

Karen told me she had no stress but continually felt under pressure and had trouble sleeping. I invited her to describe a typical day. The conversation went like this.

'When I get up in the morning I have to make breakfast for the family and get the kids off to school. As soon as everyone is out of the house I've got to race around and get the beds made. Next I tidy the kitchen and then get into the garden - I have to keep the garden tidy. Then I go to the shops and do housework and, before I know it, it's time to collect my daughter from school. I have nothing to worry about and should be happy and relaxed, but I am always in a rush, never seem to get things finished and feel under pressure.'

I encouraged Karen to substitute the phrases 'I have to' and 'I've got to' with the phrases 'I like to', 'I choose to', 'I prefer to', 'I decide to', 'I invite' and 'I allow'. At first she couldn't accept this new way of speaking. She explained to me as politely as she could

that she did have to collect her daughter and she did have to achieve tasks at home in order to play her part in the family. I reinforced that there was still a choice there - whether or not to be a good mother.

Eventually she relented and started saying things like, 'I choose to collect my daughter on time because it is important to me to be a good parent.'

By changing her language Karen began to feel considerably more in control of her life. She did confess to me that she initially felt the change was 'just words', but later her whole outlook on life softened. In most instances she did the same things - only the motivation changed. As she became more relaxed she managed to achieve more. At night she was happier and so able to sleep better.

She also took pressure off herself by using the language of permission at bedtime. She changed the words 'I must sleep' to 'I now invite sleep to come'. Consequently bedtime became more pleasurable and sleep came more easily.

Learning to relax

The ability to relax is fundamental to achieving both quality and quantity of sleep. If you are tense when you go to bed the chances are you will not be able to get comfortable and your mind will race, and sleep will be slow in arriving. When it does come you will be so wound up that you will not be able to slip into a restful and restoring sleep.

There are a number of relaxation techniques that can help you prepare for sleep. Some are designed to relax you physically and some aim to calm the mind. The two are connected, so whichever method you choose will almost certainly benefit you both physically and mentally. I have outlined my favorite techniques here, ones you can do yourself and which won't cost you any money.

There are other techniques, not listed here, that you can do during the day but they usually require professional guidance. They may work with the concept of movement and posture (yoga, t'ai chi and

Alexander technique falls into this category). Meditation is another day-time technique which enables people to be more relaxed and efficient, allowing them to sleep better at night.

Self-suggestion

A number of people have a surprising response to relaxation techniques. As soon as they hear the word 'relax', they tense up, not because they are being difficult but because they are trying so hard to relax. If this sounds like you, consider self-suggestion, an excellent method of relaxation which is also known as the autogenic method of relaxation.

Get into a comfortable position and notice any sounds that are outside the room. Allow them to be there and refocus your attention.

2 Notice any sounds that are inside the room, for example, the ticking of a clock or the sound of your own breathing.

3 Now focus your attention on your breathing. Take a deep breath in, hold it for a moment, and exhale slowly. Repeat this three times.

4 Continue to observe your breathing. Notice how it slows down and how the breaths are smooth. Remember to keep breathing throughout the exercise. Imagine you are breathing in warm air and breathing out muscle tension, so that you feel more relaxed with every breath.

5 Concentrate on feeling heaviness in your arms and legs. Say to yourself, 'My right leg is warm and heavy ... warm and heavy .. .' and work your way up through the whole body.
Progressive muscle relaxation

This technique is similar to self-suggestion. It was developed by Dr Edmund Jacobson and it is sometimes referred to as the Jacobson Technique. Follow steps 1 to 5 for 'Self-suggestion'. Then, starting with your feet, tense the muscles, hold for a few moments and then release. Always notice the difference between muscle tension and relaxation. Continue this process throughout the body. You will probably be asleep before you reach your forehead. If you aren't, finish the procedure with a visualization.

Visualization for sleep

Visualization is a wonderful technique to help sleep. It's not essential, but it helps to relax first using self-suggestion or progressive muscle relaxation. Picture yourself in the following situations as if you were looking at a movie screen, or imagine that you actually are there - it's up to you.
Hot-air balloon

Imagine a big field with a red hot-air balloon in the middle. Put all your thoughts and concerns into the balloon. Undo the ties and watch the balloon lurch into the sky, with your thoughts and concerns in it. Some people experience tingling or a feeling of lightness when they are given a holiday from their thoughts.

Secret room

In your mind's eye, take yourself to a secret bedroom which only you can go to. In this room you always feel safe and secure. Picture yourself talking around the room. Notice the decor: pictures, photographs, ornaments. Now picture yourself getting ready for bed and eventually climbing into the bed, which is clean and inviting. If life is stressful for you now, and your childhood was happy, it may be pleasant to picture yourself as a child going through these procedures.

Magic carpet

Imagine that you are lying on a magic carpet. It lifts you and takes you on a journey across deserts, mountains, oceans and cities. Take your carpet on an adventure. Explore how it feels at different heights and speeds. Try hovering over interesting buildings. Notice sounds and smells as you go. This visualization is great for people with wonderfully uninhibited and creative imaginations.

Beach scene

Take yourself for a walk along a beach. Notice the feel of the sand underfoot and the sounds of the breakers. Watch the children playing, the birds, the waves. Paddle in the water. Find a private spot among the dunes, then lie down and mold the sand to the shape of your body. Run sand through your hands. Picture yourself falling asleep.

Good sex

This needs no explanation! It works as a visualization because the storyline can be very compelling, making it easy to keep your mind away from the worries of the day.

Hypnosis

If you feel you need help with visualization, or would like to take it a step further, you might like to try hypnosis. It is very similar to visualization but the experience is considerably deeper, and is ideal for those of us who are lucky enough to have a creative imagination and an open mind. During hypnosis you will be fully aware of what is happening at all times, you are totally in control and you cannot be made to perform any action against your will. Hypnosis is a powerful technique, so if you decide to give it a go, make sure your teacher is a registered practitioner with a sound code of ethics.

Key points

• Only use your bedroom for sleep and sex.

• If you associate your bedroom with wakefulness, try spending less time in bed.

• Use permissive words like 'choose' and 'allow' instead of demanding words like 'must' and 'should'.

• Learn a relaxation technique.

Sleeping Aids

For some people the techniques described in the previous chapter are not enough, but they are reluctant to take medication. Here then are some ways to improve your sleep patterns with a little extra help.

Light

Light cannot make you sleep but it can wake you up. If you are an insomniac it is possible to use lights to reorganize your sleep patterns so that you are more alert during the day and therefore more tired and ready to sleep at night.

The nerve centers controlling our bodies' daily rhythms are stimulated by the amount of light entering the eyes. At night the pineal gland releases a hormone, melatonin, which slows down bodily processes and makes us drowsy and ready for sleep. In the morning daylight slows down the release of melatonin and we wake up.

The aim of bright light therapy is to deliver as much bright light to the back of the eye as possible. During the day, the user sits in front of a light box for around half an hour (you can read or watch TV if you want to). The bright lights suppress the release of melatonin, causing increased wakefulness. If you want to be alert in the morning and feel tired earlier at night you would use the light box in the morning. If, however, you would like to stay alert for longer into the evening you would use the light box later in the day and delay the desire to sleep. Ask your doctor for advice and help in obtaining a bright light unit.

Sound

Sound has an undeniable impact on the body. If I were to ask you to imagine the sound of fingernails scraping down a blackboard, you would probably physically shudder, but if I asked you to listen to some soothing classical music, you would most likely respond with a feeling of comfort and relaxation. On the other hand, when you need to motivate or energize yourself you may listen to music with a strong beat.

So what does this have to do with sleep? Your autonomic nervous system, which controls your breathing, heart rate and blood pressure, reacts most strongly to noise that is loud and irregular. Your body is prepared for action: adrenalin is released, blood pressure increases, pupils dilate, muscles increase in tension. Soothing noise has the opposite effect: muscles relax, the heart rate slows and the blood pressure drops - all things that signal the early stages of sleep.

If you are using noise to help you get to sleep it is important to ask yourself what response the sounds evoke in you. A colleague of mine, always a good sleeper, listens to the radio very quietly in the background. The sound of people talking engenders a feeling of company and comfort. Other people, however, might 'tune in' to the discussions and be kept awake by interesting conversation.

There are many tapes on the market which make use of noise as a sleep aid. They might use the sound of rain, running water, a purring cat, a ticking clock or breaking waves to relax and encourage sleep.

Some people respond well to the sound of background music – just make sure it is slow, relaxing music, not upbeat rock music.

Hot milky drink

Our mothers have always known that a hot milky drink will be followed by a good night's sleep. The theory was put to the test by

American sleep researcher Dr Nathaniel Kleitman, who compared the effects of a variety of foods on restful sleep. He found that people who drank Ovaltine, a malted drink made with milk, made the fewest night-time movements. Professor Ian Oswald, who runs a sleep laboratory in Edinburgh, tested the effects of Horlicks, another malted drink made with milk, on the sleep of a group of middle-aged people. On some nights he gave subjects a yellow capsule that was in fact inactive and told them it contained a 'folky' remedy for sleep; on other nights he gave them Horlicks. He found that people slept considerably better after they had Horlicks.

Some people have argued that it is the enzyme tryptophan in a milky drink that induces sleep, while others say that milk carries positive connotations of childhood. Ian Oswald, however, argues that the food value of the milk drink staves off hunger, making sleep more restful. He suggests that, while tryptophan, a natural sleep inducer, is present in dairy foods, it is in quantities too small to make a difference to the quality of sleep.

Whatever the reason, warm milky drinks before bedtime certainly help people sleep.

Ear plugs

Some people are disturbed by outside noises. Planes, traffic and neighbors can all disrupt sleep. If the external noise is persistent, ear plugs can be helpful in the short term. However, they don't enhance your sex appeal and they do make you dependent on a 'gadget'. I prefer to help people learn to sleep through noise (see pages 20-21).

I taught myself to do this years ago when I moved to a remote Scottish island to take some time out and relax. Imagine my dismay when I discovered the cottage I had rented was on the flight path for the helicopters going to the oil rigs. But I loved the cottage and decided I had to learn to live with the racket. Before long I didn't even notice the noise during the day, let alone have my sleep disrupted.

My advice is to accept the noises around you and throwaway the ear plugs.

Natural therapies

Fundamental to all natural therapies is the concept that living things are made up of structural, biological and emotional elements, and treatment must address all three elements. Some natural therapies have gained widespread acceptance in recent years, particularly acupuncture, homoeopathy and naturopathy. Be sure only to consult qualified practitioners registered with a professional body. To test whether any treatment works for you try it for two weeks and then have two weeks off. Make notes of how well you sleep and how refreshed you feel. Use the sleep management plan to help you keep track.

Food and drink

• Combat low blood sugar, which can lead to insomnia particularly if you are in the habit of eating your evening meal early, by having a mid-evening snack of slow-burning complex carbohydrates such as a slice of whole meal bread or a small bowl of pasta.

• Increase your intake of tryptophan, a naturally occurring amino acid that helps initiate sleep, by snacking on dairy products, bananas, dates and tuna in the day-time as well as during the evening.

• Warm a teapot before putting in 1 teaspoon of dried chamomile, lemon balm or lime blossom followed by 1 cup of

---

boiling water, then allow to steep for 10-15 minutes before drinking.
• Drink warm milk mixed with a teaspoon of honey before bed.

General remedies often recommended by natural therapists

Massage

A soothing massage, performed by your partner in rhythm with your breathing, can be a very relaxing experience just before bedtime and lead to a good night's sleep.

Herbal baths

An hour or so before bedtime combine several of your favorite herbs (6-8 tablespoons of fresh lavender flowers, lemon balm and rosemary leaves is a particularly soothing combination) and allow them to steep in boiling water for about 30 minutes - if using dried herbs, halve the amount. Strain them before adding to the water, and then lie back and relax.

Herbal sleep enhancers

Valerian, skullcap and passiflora are among the most effective sedative herbs. They are often combined in convenient tablet form, available from health food shops and some chemists.

Acupuncture

Acupuncture works on the principle that our bodies are traversed by a system of 12 vertical pathways called meridians. Each meridian passes through a major organ which gives the meridian its name. Ill health is viewed as the result of too much or too little energy along these meridians - in other words, the body is out of balance. The acupuncturist aims to restore balance by inserting needles on key points along the meridians. Acupressure works on the same principles, but rather than inserting needles, the therapist applies firm pressure with the fingers and thumb.

Homoeopathy

The principles of homoeopathy are similar to those of vaccines: the drug mimics the disease, and so stimulates the body's protective responses to the disease. Remedies made from animal products, minerals and plants are used. Homoeopaths say that there are no associated risks as there are with chemical medicines. The doses are so small that if the remedy doesn't work, that is all that happens – it doesn't work.

Each homoeopathic remedy is matched to the individual; when treating an ailment, such as a sleeping disorder, a homoeopath will look at the whole person. For effective prescribing you are advised to consult a registered homoeopath.

Naturopathy

Naturopathy is a common-sense approach to good health, taking the view that the body has the power to heal itself through a healthy diet, exercise and relaxation. It focuses on preventing disease rather than curing it, and views illness as a build-up of toxins or waste products, which interfere with healthy functioning - including sleep. Naturopaths claim particular success with stress and anxiety, which are at the root of many sleep problems.

After being assessed by a naturopath you will receive a program that may include advice on diet and some homoeopathic and herbal remedies to stimulate the body's healing system.

Treating yourself

With the wide array of remedies available in health-food shops and even supermarkets, self-treatment using natural therapies is tempting.

Since accurate assessment is a vital aspect of these regimes, it is advisable to consult a registered practitioner. This is especially important if you are pregnant or have a medical condition. Self assessment is very likely to be inaccurate since most of us do not have the knowledge or experience to do the job well.

Key points

• Being in bright light during the day will make you sleepier at night.

• Listening to relaxation tapes or the radio helps some people to sleep.

• Many people find a hot milky drink at bedtime helps them sleep well.

• Ear plugs, though not ideal, can be useful in the short term.

• Natural therapies can be a useful adjunct to your sleep management plan. For best results consult a registered practitioner.

Sleep Medication and Other Drugs

If lack of sleep is making a serious impact on your life, and you find that other sleep strategies aren't working for you, you may end up taking sleeping pills. Taking medication, either prescription or over the- counter (OTC), can be useful in the short term to help you sleep during a crisis - the death of a loved one, for example - but it is habit-forming. There are a number of side-effects that mean it is not a good idea to take sleeping pills as a long-term solution.

Prescription drugs

As mentioned elsewhere in this book, the best way to overcome any sleeping-related problem is to address the underlying cause. If it is necessary for you to take a prescribed medication to help you sleep, ideally you will use it to re-establish a good sleep pattern and then discard it. This is because the drug's effectiveness lessens after two to four weeks; if you become dependent on it you may be tempted to increase the dosage in order to increase your chances of sleep. There are other side-effects too: many people experience a 'hangover' the next day, dizziness and day-time drowsiness - all of which create their own set of problems, particularly in the workplace.

Another thing to consider is that sleep induced by medication is not the same as normal sleep. Drugs suppress REM sleep and deep sleep.

REM is important for mental health and deep sleep plays a vital role in physical health. Always take prescribed drugs under the conditions outlined by your doctor.

Caution: people with sleep apnoea should only take sleeping pills under the guidance of a doctor. Sleep medications, as well as alcohol and tranquillizers, depress the respiratory system, which can be quite literally fatal for people whose breathing is already affected by apnoea.

L-tryptophan

A naturally occurring amino acid that helps initiate sleep, L-tryptophan is no longer available in over-the-counter tablet form, because of a range of serious (and on occasion, fatal) side effects and a lack of research into its long-term effects. I certainly would not recommend L-tryptophan in concentrated form, but its safety is in no doubt if it is taken in its natural form, in food such as bananas, dairy products and fish.

Melatonin

This hormone, naturally occurring in the brain, is responsible for coordinating the body clock, in particular the sleep-wake cycle. It is available in tablet form in a dose many thousands of times greater than the melatonin that is naturally present in the body.

When it's time to stop taking sleeping pills

As with any prescribed medication you should seek professional advice when you want to cut down or stop taking sleeping pills. If you have been dependent on them for any length of time a sudden withdrawal can mean sleeplessness and anxiety. Interestingly, nightmares and vivid dreams can also be a problem because the amount of REM sleep (in which dreaming plays a major part) increases.

For all these reasons it is best to withdraw gradually under medical supervision while implementing the sleep management techniques described in Chapter 4. Coming off sleeping pills is challenging, and you may experience rebound insomnia because it takes a while for the brain to get used to being without the drug.

Don't assume that because you have sleepless nights you cannot do without medication. The temptation to return to the drugs is considerable, but hang on in there - things will come right eventually. If you know to expect the rebound phenomenon, you will have a greater chance of success.

It is important to get support when weaning yourself off sleeping pills in order to avoid becoming disheartened and resorting to drugs again. There are support groups for people coming off addictive medication - ask your doctor for information about groups in your area.

Over-the-counter sleeping pills

Don't imagine that just because a medication doesn't require a prescription, or comes from a natural source, it is completely safe to take. Some OTC medications are just as habit-forming as taking prescription medicine. The sleep-inducing ingredient in most of these drugs is antihistamine, which causes drowsiness, so do not use them if you are required to be active and alert immediately upon waking (for example, if you are on call for work).

However, OTC sleeping pills, also known as hypnotics, can be useful in the occasional treatment of sleeplessness.

Drugs in disguise

Drugs don't come only in medicine form - there are a number of drugs in our food and drink, and several of these have a negative impact on sleep. The most commonly used drugs are caffeine, alcohol and nicotine.

Caffeine

Probably the most widely consumed stimulant drug and the most socially acceptable; caffeine is found in coffee as well as chocolate and a number of soft drinks. Many of us consume caffeine to get an energy boost, but this is usually followed by a 'low' - a dip in performance. It is tempting to climb out of these lows by consuming another stimulant: more coffee, or a cigarette. Shift workers who struggle to keep awake at night are familiar with this phenomenon.

These manufactured highs are short-lived and if stimulants are used habitually they ultimately cause fatigue and health problems.

Coffee drinkers often have increased cholesterol levels, although it is unclear whether this is the result of the caffeine or the other chemicals found in coffee. In large doses caffeine can cause headaches, jitters and high blood pressure. Brainwave studies show that caffeine disturbs sleep most during the first three or four hours.

It delays sleep, shortens deep sleep, and reduces the overall amount of REM sleep. Coffee drinkers are groggy in the morning, which explains the need to kick-start the day with a fix of caffeine. Caffeine also decreases the effectiveness of sleeping pills, creating a temptation to increase the dose.

Table 1: Caffeine content

Coffee per cup		Soft drinks per can	
Cafetière	110–300 mg	Red Bull (250 ml)	80 mg
Filter	115–175 mg	Mountain Dew (330 ml)	54 mg
Espresso	100 mg	Diet Mountain Dew (330 ml)	54 mg
Instant	40–100 mg	Coca-Cola (330 ml)	46 mg
Decaffeinated	2–5 mg	Diet Coke (330 ml)	45 mg
		Pepsi Max (330 ml)	44 mg
Tea per cup		Pepsi (330 mg)	38 mg
1-minute brew	9–33 mg	Diet Pepsi (330 ml)	37 mg
5-minute brew	20–50 mg		

Caffeine intake recommendations

• Limit yourself to 300 mg per day (see Table).

• Avoid caffeine at least 3 hours before bedtime.

• Use caffeine strategically: have a decent, satisfying cup of coffee in the morning and switch to an alternative during the day.

• Mix decaffeinated coffee with your regular brew.

Alcohol

Alcohol is the most widely used 'sleep aid' but, although studies have shown that a little alcohol can be beneficial for your health and reduce your stress levels, it does not make a good sleeping draught.

While alcohol may help you fall asleep, it reduces the quality of sleep by making it erratic. It makes you need to get up to go to the toilet, and your body moves less during the night so that you are likely to wake in the morning with a crick in your neck or a stiff back. As the body becomes accustomed to taking in alcohol, more is needed to get the same effect. Some researchers believe that excessive alcohol intake may permanently disrupt the sleep mechanism.

Nicotine

Smokers crave nicotine both physically and mentally - this is what makes it a drug. Many smokers start smoking to help them to relax but, ironically, it has the opposite effect: nicotine is a stimulant. It is little wonder that smokers are prone to sleeplessness. The stimulant effect can make initiating sleep more difficult, and once asleep the body craves nicotine enough to wake you up. Nicotine is thought to decrease the amount of both deep sleep, which is important for physical health, and REM sleep, which helps maintain mental health.

The problem is giving up. The most important thing is the genuine desire to stop: often smokers say they hate the addiction but love the smoking. There are many books and courses and therapies, all of which claim success, but one-stop shops are rarely successful.

Smoking creates physiological and psychological addiction, so any program must address both these aspects. Most people require a multifaceted approach covering:

• how to deal with smoking triggers such as coffee, telephone, alcohol, social situations;

• how to relax both physically and mentally;

• how to deal with craving.

Key points

• Prescription and aTC sleeping pills can be useful for short term use but they are not advised for long-term use.

• Most aTC sleeping pills contain antihistamine, which causes day-time drowsiness, making them a safety hazard.

• It is essential to get the help of your doctor when coming off sleeping pills.

• Caffeine, alcohol and nicotine are drugs that can interfere with the quality of sleep.

Stress Management

One of the main reasons that people have trouble sleeping is stress.

Stress can delay sleep, break the continuity of sleep and even impair its quality. How many times have you heard someone say they can't sleep because they are worried about the mortgage or they have been churning over in their mind an argument?

Put simply, stress is an uncomfortable feeling caused by the pressures of life. Some events - relationship breakdown, for example - are acknowledged as major external stressors, but there are also internal stressors, which have to do with the way we perceive situations. Stress usually relates to conflict or unpleasant situations, but it can also be related to exciting events, such as a wedding.

Stress is normal - but the way in which we handle it has an impact not just on our sleep but on our health in general.

External stressors

Common external stressors include:

- bereavement;
- relationship breakdown;
- moving house;
- wedding;
- new job;
- exams;
- change in health;
- change in financial situation;
- time constraints.

You can often manage external stressors relatively easy by adjusting your personal circumstances. For example, if you are not happy about your situation at work you can look around for another job.

Even if the stressor is particularly difficult, such as the death of a loved one, most situations can eventually be resolved with time and the support of friends and family.

Internal stressors

Common internal stressors include:
- low self-esteem;
- lack of direction in life;

• loneliness and boredom;

• fear of the unknown, for example, illness, death, losing money, not being liked;

• perfectionism;

• feeling that you are not in control of your life;

• contained emotions, especially guilt and anger.

Internal stressors are more difficult to deal with because you cannot make them go away simply by changing what you do or by enlisting the support of your friends. You must make the change from within, which can be challenging and, for some people, threatening.

This point, that change must come from within, has been made thousands of times by the wise people of the world and yet plenty of people try to fix their internal stressors by changing partners, jobs, country or house. I call this the 'I will be happy when' syndrome: 1 will be happy when 1 have more money, I will be happy when 1 have a new car, 1 will be happy when 1 have a partner, I will be happy when my partner spends more time with me, 1 will be happy when we have a better government, I will be happy when I run my own business, I will be happy when the summer comes, I will be happy when the world is nuclear free...

People who have the '1 will be happy when' syndrome miss the point: everyone is responsible for their own thoughts, feelings and actions. No one and nothing can make you happy or unhappy without your say-so.

If you think your stressors may be internal - to do with your personality, attitudes or beliefs - ask yourself the following questions:

• What is the real issue here?
• Where does this feeling come from?
• Is the feeling useful?
• How would 1 like to be?

If you answer those four questions honestly and thoughtfully, you will have half the solution to the problem. The other half of the solution lies in the fifth question:

• What do I have to do to get there?

Stress management

Remember that stress is a normal and healthy part of life: if we never experienced stress, life could be very dull. It only becomes a problem if it is too intense or too frequent. If stress is stopping you sleeping well, effective management of stress will be part of your sleep management plan.

Ten ways to manage stress

1 Sleep well.

2 Eat a balanced diet.

3 Exercise regularly.

4 Understand and manage your thoughts, feelings and actions.

5 Continually work towards the three elements of 'hardiness': challenge, control, commitment (see below).

6 Think positively about yourself.

7 Identify and use your support networks.

8 Practice relaxation regularly.

9 Communicate honestly.

10 Allow time for yourself.

Becoming hardy

Some people have a personality characteristic known as 'hardiness', which helps protect them against the effects of stress. Hardiness consists of three main components.

• Commitment to work, family and other important issues, which helps keep difficult events in perspective.

• Control, a feeling of power over their own destiny, which means they acknowledge they may not be able to control stressful events but that they can control their response to it. They view stressful events as occasions for growth.

• Challenge, a feeling of being stretched, that their abilities are being used. What some people view as hurdles, 'hardy' people view as opportunities. A colleague of mine who was made redundant was surprised by how upset people were for her. They imagined she would be distraught, but my colleague's attitude was, 'Great - I needed a reason to leave and explore other opportunities. Without this extra push it may have been years until I took the leap. This is a blessing in disguise.'

Depression and anxiety

Depression, anxiety and insomnia almost always occur together: the problem is working out which came first. Depression and anxiety (which occur when stress gets out of control or becomes chronic) invariably cause sleep problems, but sometimes it is the other way around - it is the lack of sleep that has caused the depression or anxiety. It is important to work out which is the primary problem and manage it accordingly. Treatment of any depression or anxiety typically involves counseling, learning skills such as diaphragmatic breathing and relaxation training. Medication can help.

This outline of depressive and anxiety states may help you identify possible causes of your insomnia. If you think any of them apply to you, go to see your doctor.

Depression

We all get fed up from time to time, but if these feelings are extreme or long-lasting they may be a form of depression, which is a frequent cause of insomnia and in particular early morning awakening. There are several different types of depression, for example, after the birth of a child (post-natal depression), response to a life event (reactive depression), and overwhelming feelings of sadness or hopelessness without an obvious reason (endogenous depression).

The following description was given to me by someone who had been suffering from depression.

I was despondent, my movements and speech slowed down. I didn't know why I was alive. Sometimes I would walk in the garden, which had always given me so much pleasure, but now it just offered an escape from the house. I stopped seeing friends. I didn't feel like eating and lost weight. Cold tinned food, coffee and cigarettes kept me going. I resented the offer of help from friends: they were patronizing, I thought, why wouldn't they go away and leave me be? Sometimes I would sit and stare into space for hours.

This kind of depression is serious and debilitating. It often lasts for months, even years, and threatens marriage and jobs. If you feel you fit into this category, see a doctor immediately to discuss the many effective treatment options.

Anxiety

Like depression, anxiety can be frightening and draining. Anxiety has many forms, from a feeling of apprehension through to a fully fledged panic attack. Symptoms include pounding heart, trembling, sweating, dizziness, nausea, hot flushes, choking and an intense fear of losing control in a public place.

There are many different types of anxiety:

• Panic disorder. Extreme fear, often out of the blue, with symptoms including shortness of breath, palpitations, trembling, dizziness, tingling fingers or feet and fear of losing control.

• Agoraphobia. Literally translated, agoraphobia means 'fear of the market place'. The person avoids situations for fear of having a panic attack. Common problem situations are bridges, tunnels, shopping centers, supermarkets, aero planes (if you have a panic attack you cannot get out) and cinemas.

• Simple phobia. Extreme fear of one particular situation or object.
Simple phobias include animals, aero planes (fear of crashing), water, dentists, thunder and injections.

• Social phobia. Fear of embarrassment causes the individual to avoid other people. Common situations include eating with friends, parties, writing cheques or notes while another person is watching, and public speaking.

• Post-traumatic stress disorder. This may occur after a major traumatic event, such as an accident or physical abuse. Common symptoms include flashbacks, nightmares and emotional numbness.

• Obsessive compulsive disorder. Thoughts or actions become repetitive, like a stuck record. Usually the thoughts are punitive.

Common obsessions include repetitive checking, washing and tidying. It has been called 'doubting disease'.

• Generalized anxiety disorder. Extreme feelings of anxiety, usually associated with life events but persisting for several months.

Can medication help?

If your symptoms of depression or anxiety are so severe that you become too distressed to climb out of the situation, it is possible that medication would be useful. You may feel that counseling is useless, that the information seems puerile - or too academic, or useful for other people but not yourself - when the truth is that you have become so low that all the counseling in the world can do no good. In this situation medication can help you feel good enough to make use of counseling and take an active role in your return to health.

Key points

• Stress is a normal and healthy part of life.
• Sleep management usually involves some stress management.
• Insomnia, particularly early morning awakening, is often a mask for depression.

• If you think you are depressed or have anxiety seek professional help immediately.

Fitness and Sleep

Most people would agree that they sleep better when they are fit.

Research has shown that when fit people exercise on one day but not on another they fall asleep more quickly on the day they exercise.

What is more, athletes tend to have more deep sleep after exercise.

However, exercise immediately before bedtime makes sleep harder, so it is better not to exercise less than two hours before bedtime.

As most of us are not going to be athletes, the following guidelines are intended for ordinary people, young and old, who want to become reasonably fit with minimum effort.

Symptoms of being unfit include:

• aches and pains caused by muscle tension;
• boredom;
• lethargy/fatigue;
• muscle cramps;
• racing heart when doing everyday activities.

For many of us exercise is a chore, something that has to be done, so try picking activities that suit your lifestyle and are fun. It is important to develop and maintain regular exercise habits. Sudden bursts of strenuous exercise are to be avoided, and the older you are the more gradually you should step up your regime.

The benefits of physical fitness

Apart from improving sleep there are a number of well-documented benefits to regular exercise.
Physical benefits

• Lowers cholesterol.
• Facilitates oxygen flow throughout the body.
• Improves muscle tone and reduces muscle tension.
• Improves posture.
• Helps eliminate adrenalin from the body.
• Improves circulation and digestion.
• Improves elimination of toxins from the body (skin, digestive and respiratory system).

Psychological benefits

- Increased feeling of well-being and self-esteem.
- Increased resilience to stress.
- Increased social contact.
- Improved concentration.
- Less dependency on alcohol and drugs.

Getting fit

We all have our own view of what it means to be fit. If you can run only a few kilometers but want to be a marathon runner, by your own standards you are unfit. If, however, you can run a few kilometers but want only to be able to walk to work without getting tired, you would consider yourself fit. The question to ask yourself is, 'Am I fit enough to do what I say I want to do in my life?' If the answer is no, you are unfit.

Many of us have genuine plans to exercise but all too often we find things get in the way of our plans: it's too cold, we're too tired or too busy. I overheard a colleague comment, 'I go for a walk every Sunday, starting next week.'

In order to implement a useful exercise regime it is important to know why you are exercising and what your goals are. Take a few moments and consider the following questions:

• What do you hope to gain from an exercise regime?
• What obstacles are likely to get in your way?
• How will you get past these obstacles?
• Who can help you to achieve your goals?

Some people will want to gain the benefits of exercising without embarking on anything so daunting as a fitness regime. You may prefer to increase physical activity in your daily life by:
• walking to the shops or walking the dog;
• mowing the lawn;
• running up the stairs.

Seven rules for safe and effective exercise

Whether you decide to incorporate exercise into your everyday activities or you undertake a sport or training regime it is always necessary to consider the rules for safe and effective exercise.

1 Make exercise enjoyable

If you don't get this one sorted out, all the good intentions in the world will get you nowhere. This sounds remarkably obvious, but gymnasiums count for their profit on people who pay their subs and never attend because they don't like gyms. Many of us also have a bad relationship with expensive items of 'get fit in five minutes a day' equipment that take a prominent position in front of the television (to remind us to use them - as if we would forget) but after a while, unused, get pushed tidily under the bed. Paying a lot of money for gym membership or home exercise equipment doesn't do the trick - you do actually have to use them.

To make things fun, try exercising with others: go walking with a friend, participate in team sports, join a club, play competitively or take up a sport that comes complete with a social life.

2 Start slowly and build up gradually

When starting an exercise program start slowly and carefully, especially if you are older. Your muscle tone will gradually improve.

Exercise regularly - regular gentle exercise is safer and more effective than blasts of strenuous exercise.

3 Warm up and cool down

Warming up properly will minimize the risk of damaging your muscles. First warm up the muscles by working them gently, then do about 10 minutes of stretching, covering each group of muscles. At the end of your activity cool down by walking slowly then gently stretching again to circulate the blood throughout your body.

4 Learn to breathe properly

Some people hold their breath when making an effort. This can raise blood pressure and increase the risk of damaging the heart. During exercise try to breathe evenly and learn to breathe in through your nose and out through your mouth. Correct breathing is essential for effective exercise. Most physiotherapists and gym instructors will be able to help you with breathing. Dinah Bradley's book Hyperventilation Syndrome provides step-by-step instructions for good breathing.

5 Be gentle on muscles and joints

Jogging may be a popular exercise, but it is very harsh on the body and frequently causes injuries because of the jarring effect of feet hitting hard pavement. This problem can be helped by running on grass and wearing good-quality running shoes. Alternatively, try an activity which is gentler on the body, such as cycling, swimming or brisk walking.

6 If in doubt consult a doctor

If you are pregnant, have heart problems, become breathless, are overweight, are a smoker or have a bad back (in fact any health concerns), you should consult a doctor before undertaking any exercise program.

'No pain, no gain', the saying goes. I would like to point out that this is entirely wrong. If exercising is painful, the chances are you are damaging yourself. If you experience pain, stop the activity and consult your doctor.

7 Work on stamina, flexibility and strength

Ideally your exercise regime will include activities that improve stamina. This is done by increasing your body's capacity to utilize oxygen, which strengthens the heart and lungs. The efficient use of oxygen is essential for a well-functioning liver, and insomnia is sometimes caused by a liver being in bad shape.

Remember to exercise both sides of the body: this will help reduce aches and pains and improve posture.

Key points
• Fitness promotes good sleep, although exercise just before bedtime makes sleep harder.
• If you have any health concerns consult your doctor before changing your level of activity.
• Find a form of exercise you enjoy.
• Adhere to the principles of safe exercise: warm up properly, if you experience pain stop and consult a doctor, and learn to breathe correctly.

A Good Sleep at Any Age

Children and sleep

Most children have sleep difficulties at some stage - although the most serious problem associated with children's sleep patterns is sleep loss on the part of their parents. The most common problems children experience are nightmares and night terrors, fear of the dark and bed-wetting. As with all sleep difficulties, it is important to consider the cause of the problem before embarking on a sleep management plan.

This issue was brought home to me by a distraught mother who contacted me because her ten-year-old daughter Ruth was staying awake at night, crying and saying she was afraid of the dark. When Ruth was afraid she was allowed to sleep in her parents' bed. When her parents tried to send her back to her own bed she screamed and on one occasion she wrecked her bedroom. Understandably her parents were concerned about the cause of her fear (she wouldn't tell them what it was) and wondered if they were being cruel sending her back to her own room. They were getting tired from lack of sleep, and tempers in the whole family were wearing thin.

I decided to get to know Ruth before broaching the subject of her nighttime fears. We chatted about school, friends and family. Ruth talked about her two older brothers who were allowed, in her view, more freedom than her and received considerably more attention from her parents. She often felt left out. I commented that her bedtime behavior would have fixed that. She agreed. Further discussion revealed that in fact there were no fears - she simply enjoyed the attention she received when sleeping in her parents' bed.

When they found out the reason for Ruth's behavior, her parents made an effort to give all the children the same amount of attention.

They also learned to read better the signs of genuine night-time need. Ruth learned about the dangers of crying wolf and was encouraged to find appropriate ways to get her needs met.

When dealing with children it is not always easy to find the real cause of sleep problems because children do not have the sophisticated thought processes and language needed to communicate their desires and concerns. For this reason health professionals working with children and adolescents develop special skills to communicate with them. The use of art is popular because children may find it easier to discuss what is going on by drawing a picture to show how they feel. Parents whose children are having ongoing trouble sleeping are advised to seek help from a professional who specializes in the management of children's issues.

Bed-wetting

Most infants wet their beds as they learn to control their bladders overnight, and it is not uncommon for children up to the age of 12 to still be wetting their beds. There are different theories about the cause of bed-wetting (also called enuresis), including deep sleep and poor bladder control. Here is some advice.

• Sometimes bed-wetting can be a sign of infection. Ask your Doctor for a check-up.

• Most importantly, never get cross with your child as this will only make the situation worse. Teach the child to wash the sheets and make the bed.

• Use a buzzer and pad. The moisture-sensitive pad is placed under the sheets and the buzzer goes off as soon as it gets wet. It is hard for children to learn while they are asleep, but the loud buzzer immediately after wetting wakes the child and helps them read the messages from a full bladder.

• Sometimes a child that has been dry will start wetting the bed again after an emotional crisis. Support and comfort may be all that your child needs.

• You can wake your child during the night to take him or her to the toilet, but there is a risk that this will become a habit.

• Bed-wetting is embarrassing for children at the best of times, and it can stop them from staying at friends' houses or going on school trips. Short-term use of antidepressants can help, ensuring the child is not deprived of these activities.

Menopause and sleep

In her book A Passage to Power, Leslie Kenton states that, apart from a period of motherhood-induced insomnia which comes from having to feed a baby, the most likely time for women to have trouble sleeping is immediately before menopause. She suggests that the sleeplessness will probably come in the form of waking in the early hours of the morning. The reason for this may be the decline in levels of melatonin, which regulates the sleep-wake cycle. Hot flushes and night sweats can cause enough discomfort to disrupt sleep, in which case taking action to ease these symptoms can help.

The main message for menopausal women who have sleep disruptions is: utilize the sleep techniques outlined in this book and discuss the management of menopause-specific symptoms with a registered health professional. Ask your GP for help or contact the Family Planning Association.

Ageing and sleep

Older people don't sleep as much as younger people, but this is not because they need less sleep. They have lost the ability to sleep because their levels of melatonin (the hormone that governs the sleep-wake cycle) have reduced. They spend more time than younger people lying in bed at night trying unsuccessfully to sleep
(or without attempting sleep), and more time in bed during the day resting and napping. Sleep is more likely to be broken, deep sleep may be absent, and the restorative part of sleep, REM sleep, shifts to an earlier part of the night. The circadian rhythm (body clock) may also adjust.

Many older people adapt to these changing sleep patterns and accept the subtle changes, but for others the effects are more dramatic and lead to abnormal day-night patterns. We are what we are. Much of what we do in old age is programmed by a lifetime's habits, and our sleep patterns and practices will be affected by our previous lifestyles. It is unreasonable to expect early risers to sleep in to catch up on sleep after they retire.

It is normal for some older people to have episodes of wakefulness at night; if you return to sleep you should not consider this abnormal. If understood, the sleep changes that occur with advancing age, such as sleep loss after bereavement, can be dealt with at a personal and family level.

Older people need to be particularly careful to get enough exposure to light. Young people usually have a daily exposure to quite bright light of at least two hours, but older people generally get less than half this amount because they leave the house less often.

This reduction may well affect sleep quality. Activity during the day will also influence circadian rhythms, so a walk in the park on a sunny day will help you sleep - and is far better for your health than medication.

Sleep abnormalities may also be caused by minor physical complaints, for example, cramps in the legs and breathing problems.

Menopause can have a significant effect on the lining of the bladder tube, and the lack of estrogen makes infections more common, resulting in the need for frequent passing of urine. Hormone replacement therapy could help. Men are subject to night visits to the toilet too, often because of an enlarged prostate gland. This can be helped by drugs or surgery.

The fact is, while basic physiological changes occur in old people that will affect sleep, much of the control of sleep patterns is in your hands. Sleep disruption can be treated effectively without the use of drugs if you take a common-sense approach and get the help of a sympathetic doctor or a therapist experienced in sleep management.

Take the lead in maintaining your health and seek help sooner rather than later.

Older people and medication

Physicians tend to ask fewer questions about sleep difficulties than they do in other health areas, and when they do there is a tendency to prescribe sleeping pills. Although they may be helpful in the short term, they certainly won't help sleep long term. Some sleeping pills affect mood and the ability to concentrate and they can interact in a bad way with other drugs. The last thing an older person wants is to be taking too much medication. In principle, the fewer drugs that are taken the better.

Anyone taking more than four drugs on a regular basis should have them reviewed by their doctor at least once a year. Older people's bodies process drugs quite differently from young people's. This is because their rates of absorption and distribution through the body are different. There is, on average, less fat on a younger person's body, and their kidneys and liver work better.

Long-term use of night sedatives can have bad effects not only on sleep but also on how you feel the following day. No one wants to feel permanently hung over.

Key points

• Sleep problems can arise at any age but there are particular difficulties associated with childhood, menopause and ageing.

• It is always important to find the cause of the problem before embarking on a management plan.

• As we get older our need to sleep remains the same but our ability to sleep deteriorates.

• Sleep problems in old age can be effectively treated without the use of drugs.

Working Nights

We live in a 24-hour society. For many people this means getting up and going to work just when the rest of us are getting ready to wind down from our day's activities.

Shift workers have been hailed by Dr Marty Klein, an American shift work specialist, as the unsung heroes of society. Without them all the services that we take for granted - electricity, transportation, police and fire protection, medical care and many others - just would not function.

As any shift worker will tell you, it's not that easy to make the necessary adjustments not only to their sleeping habits, but to their whole way of life. As many as 80 per cent of shift workers complain of sleep difficulties, and these difficulties include delayed sleep, broken sleep and unrefreshing sleep. It is estimated that shift workers on average sleep two hours less per 24 hours than day workers.

The fundamental problem with shift work is that it requires you to sleep when your body wants you to be awake. The shift worker has to battle the body clock, as well as the noise and demands of family, neighbors and the world around.

Human beings are designed to be day-time creatures: we function best if we sleep at night and are active during the day. Our body clocks don't just regulate the sleep-wake cycle - to get optimum efficiency out of our bodies they control other functions too, for example, body temperature and the digestive system.

During the day our core body temperature rises in anticipation of increased activity, but at night the body cools down in preparation for sleep. Even if you are a permanent night worker this still occurs because on your days off you sleep at night and are active during the day.

The digestive juices are produced before usual daily meal times.

During the night the digestive system is on a 'go slow' and food is therefore more difficult to digest. This in part accounts for the fact that an estimated 30-40 per cent of shift workers suffer from stomach problems in the form of increased or decreased appetite, diarrhoea, constipation or indigestion. These problems may also be linked to increased caffeine intake, smoking and poor canteen facilities.

Tips for effective day-time sleep

Being able to sleep well during the day is essential to the well-being of shift workers. However, it is not recommended for anyone else to spend large amounts of the day sleeping.

• The best time to sleep is as soon as possible after the night shift. If you delay sleep your body will warm up and prepare for the day's activity.

• Ideally, have one block of sleep only.

• Most shift workers find they can only manage about three hours' sleep before their body clock or noise wakes them up. If this happens, try to have another block of sleep just before the night shift to help you stay awake at night. Two blocks of sleep are preferable to a scattered sleep pattern.

• Use black-out curtains or an eye mask. This is essential - melatonin (the hormone of sleep) is suppressed by light even when your eyes are closed.

• To minimize interruptions from the phone, use call divert, call minder, answer phone or message exchange, or turn the ring volume right down.

• Teach yourself to sleep through normal day-time noises. Failing this, use ear plugs.

Overcoming fatigue

There are nine 'switches of alertness'. Understanding these switches and how to manipulate them is the secret of gaining power over one of the most important attributes of the human brain', alertness.

Switch 1: Danger, change, interest, opportunity
Changing activity can make you more alert. This is especially effective if the body has an adrenalin rush and kicks into the flight or fight response. Keep in mind, however, that what causes an adrenalin rush one day may not another day. If you are feeling tired at work, taking a break, talking to colleagues or changing tasks can help.

Switch 2: Muscular activity
Any form of movement - even eating or talking - increases levels of alertness. If the movement is vigorous and speeds up the metabolic rate, so much the better. According to Dr Moore-Ede the effect can last for an hour or more. He makes the point that, although regular exercise is thought to promote deep sleep, which leaves you feeling more restored, it is hard to fall asleep straight after going for a jog.

Switch 3: Body clock

Your body clock will be affected by the style of roster you work. For example, a roster that rotates forwards is thought to be less fatiguing than one that rotates backwards. This is because it is more in tune with your circadian rhythms. (A forward rotation is one in which a day shift is followed by a late shift, which is followed by a night shift.) It has also been suggested that changing a roster is the most stressful thing an organization can do to its staff – organizational stress in itself causes fatigue. It is an occupational hazard that definitely has an impact on morale.

Switch 4: Light

The significance of light is one of the most researched topics in alertness studies. Bright light can be used to reset the body clock towards night-time alertness and day-time sleep (see page 26), and it can also be used to improve alertness while working, without adjusting the body clock. The intensity of the light and the length of exposure to it is the subject of much debate and research. If you want to become nocturnal, in other words invert your whole life, it is useful to use very bright light to help the body clock adapt to night times activity and day-time sleep. If, however, you want to keep your body clock oriented to day-time activity, you can use light as a night-time alerter - a short trip to a brightly lit canteen, for example, will provide enough light to alert you without adjusting your body clock.

Switch 5: Sleep

The most important fatigue management strategy is maintaining your sleep bank account in credit (restful sleep is akin to making a deposit). My own informal surveys show that many shift workers manage only four or five hours' sleep in each 24-hour period, so it is easy to accumulate a sleep debt of 15 to 20 hours a week.

Chronically sleep-deprived workers are a danger to themselves and others.

Switch 6: Food, drink and drugs

The stimulant effects of caffeine, chocolate and nicotine are well known by shift workers. However, the resulting alertness is not only short-lived, it is followed by a slump. Used regularly they cause health problems and, ironically, increase fatigue.

Some researchers have made the point that many of the health problems associated with shift work have more to do with the increased caffeine and nicotine consumed by shift workers than the shift work itself.

There has been a suggestion that food that is rich in carbohydrate (potatoes, rice, pasta) promotes sleep, and food that is rich in protein (meat, eggs, dairy products) promotes wakefulness. The research in this area is inconclusive, however, and I recommend carbohydrate during the night shift, especially after midnight. This is because the digestive system is on 'go slow' and protein is hard to digest.

Instead of coffee or tea, drink hot water, cordial, fruit juice or soup.

Switch 7: Sound

Many organizations use sound as an alerter. Continuous background noise and white noise cause fatigue, but loud music and radio shows can help you be alert.

Switch 8: Odor

Although there has not been a great deal of interest from the scientific community in the use of odor as an alerter, many people are aware of the 'Wake up!' effect of some smells, for example, perfume. Some nurses find cleaning their teeth with mint toothpaste during the night shift helps keep them alert.

Switch 9: Temperature

There is a great temptation for night staff, especially those who work in control rooms, to create a warm, cozy environment, but this only promotes sleepiness. Warmth causes fatigue and cold causes alertness; very cold temperatures, however, create fatigue because the body is working hard to keep warm.

Clearly these switches of alertness need to be adapted according to your work requirements and personal preferences. What works for you one day may not another day. What works for one organization may be inappropriate for another.

When choosing which to use, ask yourself the following questions:

• Is it tried and tested by shift workers?
• What is the scientific view?
• How will it affect my health and safety in the short and long term?
• Will it create other problems?
• How will the strategy be viewed by my colleagues and managers?

Professional help from a consultant will help your employer make appropriate choices that benefit both you and the organization.

Power naps

The use of a short nap is recognized as an alerter. Most researchers recommend no more than 20 minutes to ensure that you do not sink into a state of deep sleep. Waking up after a short sleep usually takes only a few seconds, but if you do go into deep sleep you are likely to wake up feeling groggy and the recovery time is much longer.

Many organizations do not allow napping because they think it unprofessional or a waste of company time. Controlled napping is, in fact, very professional because there is no doubt it enhances performance and safety. Perhaps organizations should introduce strategic napping for pilots as a way of improving crew alertness and safety.

Key points

• Shift workers have special problems getting enough good quality sleep.

• Improve daytime sleep by going to bed as soon as the shift ends, using black-out curtains or an eye mask, and turning off the phone.

• Train yourself to sleep through noise.

• Use the switches of alertness to keep you awake at work.

The 7 Habits of Highly Effective Sleepers

I have already suggested that many sleep problems are the result of poor sleep habits. The assumption is that if we learn poor sleep by developing a bad habit we can also learn good sleep by learning useful habits. As children we had many invaluable skills that, with the responsibilities and pressures of adulthood, we have lost. As adults we need to relearn the habits that as children we adopted instinctively.

Steven R. Covey, author of the best-selling The 7 Habits of Highly Effective People, defines a habit as the intersection of knowledge, skill and desire. Knowledge is about what to do and why, skill is about how to do it, and desire is the motivation to do it. In order to make something a habit, he argues, we need all three. He suggests that a habit is a 'consistent and often unconscious pattern of behaviour'.

Following is a list of habits associated with good sleep. Each habit means something different to each person. I have invited my colleagues and patients to comment on the habits. Not every habit works for every person. Read through the list and decide which ones you want to adopt, and note them in your sleep management plan

Habit 1: Choose to let go

Bedtime is a time for rest and sleep, not ruminating, worrying or planning. The duvet is the last frontier: if you can't get away from pressures of life when you are in bed, then relaxed sleep is not possible. It is essential to be able to let go at bedtime.

I am a doctor at a busy accident and medical clinic. During the day I see all types of trauma and so often real sadness. For me letting go means leaving all work-related thoughts at work. I always leave my uniform at work and when I leave the clinic I remind myself that I did the best I could and everything is now out of my hands. Some people might think this is harsh but in reality, in order for me to be the very best I can be for my patients, I must truly take time out, rest properly and sleep properly.

I run my own business and there is always something to think about: staff, money, supplies, marketing. It is never-ending. Sometimes I lie in bed thinking about all the things J should do. For me letting go means writing comprehensive lists of tasks for myself. Once it is written I don't need to think about it any more. I can let go of all the busy thoughts.

I have been having problems in my marriage recently. For a while I would think about what happened. My mind would go round and round going over what he said, what I said - could I have saved the situation? For me letting go meant keeping my thinking and planning as a daytime activity. I went to a marriage guidance counselor and I know that whatever the outcome I will have done everything I can. Yes - letting go means sorting out troubles in the daytime so I can truly let go of them at night-time.

For me letting go means making sure that I can rest in my bed at night with a clear mind. I have to confess that this hasn't always been easy. Last year I let a friend down badly; I knew I had upset him and I felt guilty about my behavior. Eventually I visited my friend to apologize and put things right. I think it is important to deal with mistakes and then move on. I am not sure if my friend has forgiven me but I know that I have done everything I can to make amends. Ruminating and inflicting myself with further guilt will not help the situation. I can now let go.

Habit 2: Limit the toxins

Alcohol, nicotine and caffeine are probably the most commonly consumed toxins. Good sleepers are aware of the impact these have, not just on sleep but on health in general. Don't forget that sleeping pills are included in this category.

I was a keen coffee drinker - it was definitely a habit. I didn't drink coffee because I really wanted or needed it - I drank it because it was there, and because I liked having a hot drink in my hand to sip at. Now I have one good cup of coffee per day and drink hot water the rest of the time. Hot water achieves the same result. Reducing my caffeine has increased my energy and improved my sleep.

Coming off sleeping pills was a challenge. My sleep did get worse before it improved. i worked on the 7 Habits and slowly, with the help of my doctor, reduced my medication. I can't say it was easy. For a while the habits were interesting theories to me but I hadn't incorporated them into my subconscious - I wasn't 'walking the talk'. I had seven new theories and fewer pills: this was scary. Not surprisingly my sleep became worse before it improved. A couple of times I was so tired from sleep loss that I was crying. It was very tempting to return to the medication just to get one good night's sleep. I think that the strong support of my doctor and my wife pulled me through. All I can say is that to be prepared is to be forewarned.

A year later I no longer take medication and the 7 Habits have flowed into other areas of my life. To my surprise there were additional spin-offs. My advice to anyone coming off medication is to work with a health professional, be prepared for the feeling of withdrawal, and work with the 7 Habits every day. Make sure they are real and not just interesting information.

Habit 3: Work towards fulfillment

People who feel fulfilled in life usually go to bed with a feeling of satisfaction. Satisfaction is equated with good sleep. They know who they are, what they are doing and why they are doing it. Some people go through life with positive direction while others need support. Those who lack direction are likely to be poor sleepers.

Some time ago I sought help for my sleep. At the interview I was asked if! was fulfilled in my life. I answered, 'Yes, totally.' I was a busy executive with a high-profile organization. I had everything

I thought I wanted: status, career prospects, high income and a family. But the question played on my mind - I kept asking myself if this was really what I wanted. Something inside me said no. However I didn't know what I did want.

I decided to make a start by exploring my own desires and aspirations, asking myself what really mattered. I enlisted the help of a counselor; I read books, talked to friends and took some long walks on the beach. I came to some startling conclusions. What I really wanted was to see more of my family, plan my own time and enjoy quality friendships. I did not really want to work my way up the corporate ladder and receive a gold watch at the end.

I gave up my career a year ago. I now develop houses for a living and I spend a great deal more time with my family - we go sailing with friends and life is so much easier. I feel in charge of my life. It goes without saying that the happier I felt, the better I slept.

I knew that I didn't feel fulfilled in my life. This embarrassed me because I was a full-time mother, the most important job in the world, so I should feel fulfilled. I think the problem was that I spent all my time looking after other people's needs and my own personality never had time to emerge.

One day I woke up and decided that this was my life so I should make it a good one. I signed on at the local college to study carpentry, of all things. Now I take great pride in making furniture and knowing that I have done a good job. As soon as I started the course I felt like somebody. I felt a better person, my spirits lifted, and I am sure that I became a better mother. I have felt better in all areas of my life since becoming a student – my health and motivation have improved. I am more comfortable and relaxed with myself and I sleep better.

Habit 4: Relax

You only need to use the necessary muscles to do a job, but most of us use many more. We frown while we are writing, we jiggle our feet while we are speaking on the phone, we tense our shoulders while we are driving.

When we overuse muscles they become constantly tense, knot up, release toxins and cause discomfort. This may result in headaches, shoulder pain and general muscle tension. Some people have been in this state of heightened physical tension for so long that it becomes the norm. People who are physically tense are probably also mentally tense, which is a recipe for poor sleep.

When I was a teenager I damaged my back. The pain caused me to tense the muscles on one side. You can imagine the tension and pain made sleeping very difficult. Sometimes just turning over would give me stabs of pain and I would wake up. This could happen four or five times in a night. Eventually I took up yoga.

This was the best thing I had ever done. The stretching movements were great for my back, and I learned relaxation. After a while my muscles became more balanced, the pain decreased and my sleep improved.

My husband was a poor sleeper, probably because - he would hate to admit it - he didn't handle stress well. This was obvious to me when he was driving his car and he got infuriated with other road users. The language was terrible, and he scowled, clenched his jaw and hunched his shoulders. He learned a relaxation technique and had to apply it to activities of daily living such as driving. Not only has he learned new ways of reacting physically, he has learned new ways of thinking. He copes better in the car, is more at ease with difficult situations and, of course, is sleeping better.

Habit 5: Don't think about sleep

It's simple: people who sleep well do not go to bed wondering if they are going to sleep well. It is a foregone conclusion. Perhaps it is the absence of wondering that does the trick.

I am sure this is correct. I am a good sleeper: I enjoy going to bed.

I can sleep anywhere, any time. When I think about it, I would say it is something to do with the way we were brought up. Our parents were very positive. They taught us to believe in ourselves, to believe we were happy, healthy and able to enjoy a useful life.

Sleep as such was never mentioned, I suppose because it is part of life. This positive outlook was a way of life and in my opinion it was a habit I was taught at an early age.

I used to go to bed wondering if I would sleep. I am sure other people don't do that. My sleep improved when I started to behave like a good sleeper. In other words, I stopped thinking about sleep. If I woke in the night I didn't let it worry me and I never discussed my sleep patterns with other people. Getting away from the subject of sleep worked for me.

Habit 6: Maintain good self-esteem

People who have a good sense of self-worth usually go to bed feeling they have had a good day in which they enjoyed interactions with other people. When our self-esteem is challenged or eroded, stress symptoms are likely to develop, especially if the problem has been going on for years.

I always used to feel good about myself. Lately I have been unhappy about my looks. Ageing and gravity is taking its toll. I feel young on the inside but am dismayed every time I look in the mirror. This has started to affect my sleep. Eventually I decided to stay as I am and grow old gracefully, accepting myself as I am - easy to say but harder to do. Reinhold Niebuhr's serenity prayer helped: 'God grant me the serenity to accept the things I cannot change, the courage to change the things I can, and the wisdom to distinguish one from the other.' I realized I was spending hours worrying about the effects of getting older. I needed to accept the ageing process. I know full well the saying 'whatever you focus on expands'. I was focusing on the negative aspects of ageing. It is not surprising that my confidence and sleep deteriorated. Acceptance was the only way.

I started focusing on the benefits of ageing such as increasing character (which I love) and the ability to do whatever I wanted to, regardless of what other people thought. Some people would call me eccentric but I like that too. Sleep - yes, it has improved.

Mainly because I like myself better - less stress, more sleep!

Habit 7: Address unresolved issues

Many of us have troubles that have never been dealt with adequately, events that have left us with feelings of guilt, anger, upset, hurt or fear. These feelings follow us around everywhere we go, coloring every interaction.

I didn't feel wanted as a child. I think the feeling of being unwanted is so familiar to me that it crops up repetitively even today. Events that other people seem to brush off I am likely to interpret as a form of rejection - like the time my best friend forgot to come to my party and the time I asked a woman out and she said no. Now I go to great lengths not to be rejected - I just don't put myself at risk. I hate being turned down. I feel jealous of other people at times because everyone has more fun than I do.

I don't sleep well - I never have and I probably won't until I drop some of the upsetting events from my childhood and lead a full life today.

I was a victim as a child and I still am in many ways. I was afraid of my father and I couldn't wait to leave home. I was married by the age of 19 and pregnant soon after. I depended on my husband for money to buy the groceries and pay the bills. On payday he would gamble or drink his wages away. I started going to the casino and pleading with him to give me his pay packet. We had a family to feed. When he got home ... well you can guess the rest.

Sleep? No I didn't sleep well, mainly because of worry and fear.

The odd thing is, I never realized I was entitled to something better. At the time I thought that I deserved what was happening.

Eventually I left my husband and found a flat on my own. I started seeing a counselor who discussed repetitive cycles. It is so obvious to me now that I had learned to be a victim and repeated that style in my marriage. I learned about my rights as a human being, attended assertiveness courses and little by little took charge of my life. Parts of this were scary because one of the trade-offs of being a victim was that I could blame other people for the problems in my life. Now I am responsible for everything.

This made me nervous at first and my sleep became worse, but after a few months I became more comfortable and my sleep improved.

I should point out that the old feelings have never really gone away. When they come up I laugh at them and see them as a habit, a habit I can choose not to act on.

Your Sleep Management Plan

The most important thing about improving your sleep patterns is figuring out why you are not sleeping. Take some time now and consider the things you are doing right, and the areas you might be able to improve. Write down the things you may need to help you, for example, books, courses, counseling. Remember that good sleep is about what you do in the daytime as well as what you do at night.

Which of the 7 Habits do you want to develop?

- Habit 1: Choose to let go.
- Habit 2: Limit the toxins.
- Habit 3: Work towards fulfillment.
- Habit 4: Relax.
- Habit 5: Don't think about sleep.
- Habit 6: Maintain good self-esteem.
- Habit 7: Address unresolved issues.

	What I do now that works	Areas for improvement	Resources
Bedroom environment			
Thoughts and attitudes			
Stress			
Communication skills			
Family/social life			
Physical health			
Mental health			
Exercise			
Diet			
Relaxation skills			

Sleep diary

To help you assess your sleep progress, keep a record of your sleep patterns. Note the times when you take medication or drink coffee, tea and alcohol, to see if they affect your sleep.

WEEK 1	Mon	Tue	Wed	Thu	Fri	Sat	Sun
Total hours asleep							
Bedtime							
Final morning awakening							
Time taken to fall asleep							
Length of awakenings							
Medication (time & quantity)							
Coffee/tea (time & quantity)							
Alcohol (time & quantity)							

Strategies used:

Observations:

WEEK 2	Mon	Tue	Wed	Thu	Fri	Sat	Sun
Total hours asleep							
Bedtime							
Final morning awakening							
Time taken to fall asleep							
Length of awakenings							
Medication (time & quantity)							
Coffee/tea (time & quantity)							
Alcohol (time & quantity)							

Strategies used:

Observations:

WEEK 3	Mon	Tue	Wed	Thu	Fri	Sat	Sun
Total hours asleep							
Bedtime							
Final morning awakening							
Time taken to fall asleep							
Length of awakenings							
Medication (time & quantity)							
Coffee/tea (time & quantity)							
Alcohol (time & quantity)							

Strategies used:

Observations:

WEEK 4	Mon	Tue	Wed	Thu	Fri	Sat	Sun
Total hours asleep							
Bedtime							
Final morning awakening							
Time taken to fall asleep							
Length of awakenings							
Medication (time & quantity)							
Coffee/tea (time & quantity)							
Alcohol (time & quantity)							

Strategies used:

Observations: